ALTERNATIVE

FIRST AID

REFERENCE GUIDE

FOR CAMPERS, PREPPERS, AND

HOUSEHOLD USE

By Kerri Rivera and John Thomas

Alternative

First Aid Reference Guide

for Campers, Preppers, and Household Use

ISBN: 979-8-3305-0675-0

MEDICAL DISCLAIMER

The information presented in this book is not intended or implied to be a substitute for professional medical advice, diagnosis or treatment. All content, including text, graphics, images and information contained in this book is for general information purposes only. Kerri Rivera and John Thomas make no representation and assume no responsibility, legal or otherwise, for the accuracy of information contained in this book. Books are a snapshot in time, and the information this book contains is subject to change as new research becomes available. You are encouraged to confirm any information obtained from or through this book with other sources. Please review all information regarding any medical condition or treatment with your physician. You are ultimately responsible for your own choices surrounding your health and the health of your children.

FINDING THE INFORMATION YOU NEED

The Table of Contents will help you find frequently used sections such as "Instructions for Making CD." Chapter 7 lists treatments for a long list of health conditions and describes treatments for specific parts of the body.

If you don't find the information you are seeking in the Table of Contents, then please use the detailed List of Topics in this Book, which follows immediately after the Table of Contents.

Since this is a short book, most people will benefit by reading it through from cover to cover to get an overview of the treatment options that are available. At that point, the book will become a reference that you can use over and over again to find the bits of information you need for the specific situations you are facing.

"Are you ready to learn the truth about the future of health and healing? Neither should be as complicated or as costly as we have been led to believe."

Kerri Rivera

TABLE OF CONTENTS

LIST OF TOPICS IN THIS BOOK

Zeolite, 90

KERRI RIVERA'S WEBSITES

Kerri Rivera – Real Solutions

https://www.kerririvera.com/

This website contains large amounts of free information that will help you on your journey to better health. Even though much of the information speaks to autism recovery, the truth is that the recovery process for autistic children and adults is not that different from the process we all need to follow as we seek to overcome the causes of chronic illness, which are primarily inflammation and toxicity.

CD Autism – Kerri Rivera

You can buy books here:

https://cdautism.org/

Kerri Rivera's Newsletter

https://www.kerririvera.com/newsletter./

CONTACT KERRI RIVERA

Ask Kerri a Question

If you or someone you know would like additional instructions on how to use the suggestions in this book or you need guidance for other health challenges, then you should feel free to contact Kerri.

Questions can be sent to her by email:

Email: kerri@kerririvera.com

Consultations with Kerri

If you wish to speak with Kerri, then send an email to Kerri with your request. She will describe the consultation process and the charges for this service.

INTRODUCTION

Whether the health challenges you face are acute or chronic – minor or life-threatening, you will find helpful suggestions in these pages.

The treatments described here are part of what is now known as the "CD Protocol" developed by Kerri Rivera. CD refers to chlorine dioxide, ClO2. Chlorine dioxide is the center pin of the CD protocol, but it is only one of several key ingredients used in the pharmacy of the future that will be described in these pages.

First Aid Comes First

This is a first aid reference. It is intended to provide basic information that will help people start down the road towards healing. It does not contain comprehensive discussions of scientific and medical research. Such discussions are contained in Kerri Rivera's larger book that will be published later in 2020, and also made available on her websites. Her websites contain videos, weekly newsletters, books, and testimonies. See the page that lists Kerri Rivera's websites, which preceded this introduction.

More than an Autism Researcher

Kerri Rivera has gained worldwide recognition over the past ten years for her work with autistic children. Her CD protocol has helped more than 800 children recover from autism.

Even though the CD protocol was developed for autism treatment, many other people have adopted some or all of it for treating dozens of other kinds of illnesses.

Initially, it was the parents of autistic children who started using the CD protocol for their own health problems after seeing the powerful results it achieved for their children. As word spread, chronically ill people who were poorly served by the conventional medical care system began experimenting with the protocol for their health problems as well.

Many chronically ill people have spent hundreds of thousands of dollars going from doctor to doctor and from pharmaceutical drug to pharmaceutical drug with little or no benefit. They turned to the CD protocol with a desperate hope of receiving help. Fortunately, many who tried it were thrilled with the positive changes in their lives.

The CD protocol is a powerful tool for those who are open minded and who have come to realize that the conventional medical care system does not always have a helpful answer for every person's health challenges.

Conditions Treated by the CD Protocol

The following list is not exhaustive. It identifies the major problems that the CD protocol has been used to address. This book will not go into a detailed discussion of each problem, but it will provide a beginning point for those seeking help for what ails them.

Some problems are acute such as the common cold and ear infections. Some problems are life-threatening such as malaria. Some problems are chronic and epidemic in their frequency such as Lyme disease and diabetes.

Here is the list: MRSA, malaria, dengue, diabetes, fungus, viral issues, bacteria related illnesses, parasitic infections, tumors, cysts, cold, flu, candida, conjunctivitis, ear infections, diarrhea, constipation, hemorrhoids, high blood pressure, stroke, cancer, Lyme, autism, prostate, sinus infection, UTI, fibromyalgia, hepatitis (A-B-C), eczema, psoriasis, Crohn's, abscess.

International Network of CD Researchers

Kerri Rivera does not claim to have developed the one and only chlorine dioxide protocol – in fact, she respectfully acknowledges the work of many other chlorine dioxide researchers, because together they are pursuing a common goal.

Each researcher is providing healing alternatives that will help to address specific aspects of the weakened and sickened condition of humanity. In short, they are all working to use simple and inexpensive methods to save the human race from declining health, which, if left unchecked, will result in massive disability and death for millions of men, women, and children around the world.

Opposition to Chlorine Dioxide

As you might expect, chlorine dioxide researchers and those who recommend the use of chlorine dioxide experience intense opposition.

Big Pharma is leading the attack against Kerri Rivera and many other high-profile CD researchers. In large part, those who oppose CD research hate the fact that it is promoting the use of highly effective, non-patentable, and inexpensive treatments.

Big Pharma and the conventional medical establishment know that if they don't protect their expensive drugs and their expensive procedures, their treatments will eventually be replaced by simple, effective and inexpensive alternatives. Thus, they are engaged in a fierce battle to maintain market share and to preserve their costly medical treatment facilities.

As a result, a massive propaganda campaign is being implemented through mainstream media and the internet. The goal is nothing less than the total discrediting of CD researchers including Kerri Rivera.

This means that when you see Kerri Rivera's name and her research being dragged through the mud on mainstream network TV news programs, in nationally known newspapers, and on the internet, it is because her work is successful, and the opposition is feeling threatened. They are doing everything they can to destroy Kerri Rivera's reputation – and not just her, but anyone who is promoting alternatives to pharmaceutical based medicine.

Censored and Economically Attacked

The work of Kerri Rivera is not just being criticized, but also censored with the hope of destroying her economic capacity to continue.

Amazon took down her previous book on the CD protocol and autism treatment from its website in February of 2019. YouTube purged Kerri's videos from its website in March of 2019. Facebook purged her original groups in March of 2018 and finished off the process by removing the rest of Kerri's groups in May of 2019. Yahoo deleted her account in April of 2019. eBay removed listings to anything that contained her name in May of 2019. Vimeo took down her video account in June of 2019. Instagram took down her account in August 2019.

Google changed their algorithms in June of 2019 to hide positive information about alternative health, which resulted in only negative information about Kerri's work being shown.

PayPal closed her account in June of 2017 preventing her from receiving money for product sales. Authorize.net took down her account in July of 2018 preventing her from receiving credit card transactions.

The Truth is Still being Revealed

This slender book represents a renewal of the effort to disclose the truth about the CD protocol and to make it even more accessible. It does not describe every piece of the CD protocol, because its focus is first aid – a beginning point for healing.

It is alternative first aid for those who have come to appreciate the body's innate ability to heal – more than they appreciate the options currently being sold by conventional medical services and Big Pharma.

It is intended to be a first aid reference for preppers, campers and anyone who wants simple and effective healthcare alternatives they can freely use at home.

A Portable Pharmacy for the 21st Century

If you were going on a camping trip, preparing for unexpected events, or simply creating a little pharmacy of the future at home, then these are the five items that you would want to have for your immediate use.

- Kit for making CD

- DMSO

- Bentonite clay

- Black seed oil

- Gravity fed water purification system. (You would want a water purification system that does not require electricity or pressurized water to produce water free of toxins.)

Each Remedy is Important

As you read through this book you will quickly realize the book emphasizes the use of CD. This is because of CD's universal capacity to restore health.

This should not be taken to mean that the other remedies are less important. Each has its specific and important uses.

Detailed Overview of the CD Protocol

If you would like to view a detailed presentation on the entire CD protocol, then please watch Kerri Rivera's video presentation prepared for AutismOne. It discusses many topics other than autism.

Go to:
https://www.kerririvera.com/

Scroll down to the video link entitled:

Kerri Rivera's Autism Protocol Video – AutismOne 2019 or the most recent year

CHAPTER 1: CHLORINE DIOXIDE

Chlorine dioxide (ClO2) is a yellow-green gas. It was discovered in 1814. Since the early 1900s, people have been using it as a disinfectant.

Chlorine dioxide, also known as CD, is used to disinfect food and surgical tools. It is sprayed on produce before it goes to market. It can sterilize air and improve air quality. CD is more effective than hydrogen peroxide for killing bacteria. [3]

Chlorine dioxide has been approved by the US Federal Drug Administration (FDA) for use on food and for disinfecting water. It also has been approved by the US Environmental Protection Agency (EPA) and endorsed by the World Health Organization (WHO) for water purification. [1] Chlorine dioxide research shows that it is clearly not harmful to human life. [2]

The Great Bleach Lie

Chlorine dioxide is not bleach! Chemically, chlorine dioxide (CLO2) and Sodium hypochlorite, bleach, (NaOCl or NaClO) are two distinctly different chemicals.

Let me say this in another way. Chlorine dioxide kills pathogens on food and in the human body with oxygen. Yes, the same oxygen we breathe every day to live.

Sodium hypochlorite (bleach) kills pathogens with chlorine.

During World War I, chlorine gas was used as a weapon to disable and kill allied soldiers. It was released into the air and it flowed down into the trenches where soldiers were positioned. [3] Chlorine gas is highly destructive to life [3], but this is **not** the case with chlorine dioxide. [4]

If a person is opposed to using or consuming substances that contain chlorine, then they should also be opposed to using table salt. Plain old table salt (NaCl) contains sodium and chlorine. They are bonded together to form a substance that is absolutely essential for life. The human body knows what to do with tiny amounts of chlorine from salt and uses it for many purposes including the production of hydrochloric acid (HCl) in the stomach, which is required for digesting the food we eat.

It is true that chlorine dioxide is used in paper making as a whitening agent, however that does not mean that it is bleach. So, any time you hear somebody refer to chlorine dioxide as "industrial bleach," then you know they are being intentionally deceptive or are simply misinformed by those who seek to discredit the use of CD.

Family of Pro-Oxidants

CD is one of four pro-oxidants. Bleach is not a member of the family — not even a close cousin.

The four members of the pro-oxidant family are:

Chlorine dioxide (CD) 0.95 volts

Oxygen 1.30 volts

Hydrogen peroxide 1.80 volts

Ozone 2.07 volts

The human body is approximately 1.28-1.30 volts. This means that CD is very safe, because its voltage is lower than the voltage of the body and therefore will not harm cells or tissues. Even though it cannot harm the body, its voltage is high enough to kill pathogens. This is why CD is such a safe and potent remedy.

CD also assists with heavy metal detoxification. It is not a chelator. But it makes toxic metals in the body available to chelators that are being used at the same time as CD.

Powerful Functions of CD

CD is antibacterial, antifungal, antiviral, and anthelminthic. It reduces inflammation and helps reduce the heavy metal burden in the body.

CD can go through bacteria cell membranes and cause their death. In labs it deactivates fungal spores. It damages the cell walls and it causes the toxins, the mold, the candida, or the bacteria to basically ooze itself to death.

Since CD is a gas, it can easily penetrate and disintegrate pathogens throughout the body. It is not limited by the blood brain barrier, vascular system, or the GI tract. Thus, when a person drinks it, it travels throughout the body.

Oxidants and Antioxidants

There is a lot of attention given to antioxidant substances. So much attention that one might assume that anything that is not an antioxidant is dangerous. But, antioxidants cannot perform the oxidizing function.

The human body needs both antioxidants and oxidants. They each perform different positive functions for our bodies. CD is an oxidizing agent.

CD gains electrons during chemical reactions as it interacts with compounds in the cells of pathogens. When CD takes electrons from microbes, the microbial bonds weaken and the cell breaks apart, thus causing cell death for the microbe. This is the power of an oxidizing agent such as CD. This is not a dangerous process to the body, but a process that brings healing to a body that is overwhelmed by pathogens. As a pro-oxidant, chlorine dioxide does not cause oxidative stress. It reduces oxidative stress by killing the pathogens that cause the oxidative stress.

Your Doctor's Opinion about CD

It is not likely that the typical physician has any knowledge of CD. If you talk to your doctor about chlorine dioxide, your doctor is likely to hear "chlorine," associate it with swimming pool chemicals and say you should avoid it. If your doctor shows no willingness to do a little research to learn both sides of the story, then you might do well to change doctors.

The internet still has both positive and negative views of chlorine dioxide. However, the new filters being used against alternative healthcare options by Google are distorting the truth about CD. Thus, it will be necessary to use a different search engine when researching CD.

Methods of Use – (See Chapter 6)

See Chapter 6: Using CD, for detailed instructions for making and using chlorine dioxide.

References

[1] "Parents Seeking Non-Medical Help for Autism Online Being Reported to CPS to Have Children Medically Kidnapped," Health Impact News, 6/3/2019.

https://healthimpactnews.com/2019/parents-seeking-non-medical-help-for-autism-online-being-reported-to-cps-to-have-children-medically-kidnapped/

[2] Judith R. Lubbers, Sudha Chauhan, and Joseph R. Bianchine; "Controlled Clinical Evaluations of Chlorine Dioxide, Chlorite and Chlorate in Man," Fundamental and Applied Toxicology, 1981. https://www.sciencedirect.com/science/article/pii/S0272059081800425

[3] "Was Chlorine Gas Used in World War 1?" Answers.com Retrieved 6/20/2019. https://www.answers.com/Q/Was_chlorine_gas_used_in_world_war_1

[4] "Kerri and Dr Seneff June 11 2019 CD cures Autism," YouTube. https://www.youtube.com/watch?v=u3ek5Ly1KmI

CHAPTER 2: DMSO

DMSO or dimethyl sulfoxide is an organic sulfur compound. It is a by-product of the paper making industry where pure cellulose is extracted from wood chips for making paper.

Its medical properties were discovered in 1963 by a research team headed by Stanley W. Jacob, MD. [1]

Powerful Functions of DMSO

People use DMSO for hundreds of ailments including pain, strokes, and cancer treatment. It can be purchased online and in some health food stores or even from some conventional pharmacies.

DMSO is the best solution for pain – be it acute or chronic. It is highly effective for the relief of inflammation which leads to pain. It also works as a curative solution to the causes of pain.

It is great for back pain from strains, and for the discomfort and pain of monthly menstruation.

The uses of DMSO, however, go far beyond pain. It is used as an anti-cancer agent and as a treatment against pathogens.

Safety Facts

DMSO has FDA approval for use as a preservative of stem cells, bone marrow cells, organs for transplant, and is approved for interstitial cystitis –

a painful inflammatory condition of the bladder which is very difficult to treat with other therapies. [1]

"It is safe to declare that DMSO is among the safest substances in the world today." [1]

Methods of Use

DMSO can be taken orally with water, used on the skin as a transdermal agent, and can be given intravenously.

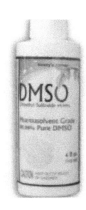

Warning: DMSO should NEVER BE USED IN AN ENEMA. The reason for this warning is linked to the ability of DMSO to penetrate tissues and cells, and to take other substances with it as it travels. You wouldn't want DMSO to drive toxic substances that are in the colon into the membranes and muscles of the colon walls.

For most situations, when applying DMSO to the skin, the 99.9% pure DMSO can be used without diluting it with water. If you will be using it on the neck, head, or genitalia you should add water to the DMSO so it does not irritate sensitive skin.

When applying it on the skin of knees or hips where arthritis pain is common, it can be applied straight from the bottle on clean skin.

There is no limit to the amount of DMSO that can be applied to the skin. There is also no limit to the frequency of using it on the skin.

When taking DMSO orally, we can take up to 25 ml per day. It should be mixed with clean filtered water before swallowing. It should not be taken with food. It is best to divide the dose into three parts and to spread the doses out over the day.

It is always a good idea to start with a small dose such as 1 ml of DMSO in water and work up to larger doses over 20 days until you reach a full dose. This will avoid possible detoxification reactions which could include "stomach upset, headaches, dizziness, and sedation." [1]

As mentioned, DMSO has the ability to drive other substances into tissue. It is great for driving CD into the skin. Do this by spraying CD on the skin and then apply some drops of DMSO on top of the CD.

In the case of breast cancer, lumps, tumors, or anything suspicious under the armpit region, it is a good idea to apply DMSO to the area after showering. Wait about 5 minutes until it has dried, then dress.

Measuring DMSO and Mixing it in Water

Never measure DMSO in a plastic spoon or use a plastic cup for mixing DMSO with water, because it can leach toxic chemicals from the plastic. Always use a glass container for mixing.

Only Apply to Clean Skin

DMSO will take anything through the skin. So, it is very important to only use clean hands to apply it to clean skin. Other than that, you cannot go wrong. Of course, if you take it orally you might be told that you smell like garlic or onions – a little garlic aroma is a very minor inconvenience when compared to serious illness. The smell that can be detected around the body is caused by the high sulfur content of DMSO, which is also found in garlic and onion.

If you want to avoid the aroma, then just use it topically or take oral doses of MSM (Methylsulfonylmethane). MSM functions similarly to DMSO for addressing pain and inflammation.

Reference

Gabriela Segura, M.D., "DMSO – The Real Miracle Solution," Health & Wellness, Sott.net, 5/12/2011.

CHAPTER 3: BENTONITE CLAY

Bentonite clay has strong ionic properties, which enables it to attract and bind together with heavy metals, pathogens, and many types of toxins including mycotoxins (from mold). If it is taken orally, the bentonite clay holds the undesirable substances until they are eliminated from the body. If used topically on the skin as in a bath, then the undesirable substances are drawn out of the body.

Powerful Functions of Bentonite Clay

Bentonite clay has the unusual property of being able to both adsorb and absorb harmful substances. When it adsorbs substances, it causes them to stick to the surface of the clay particles. When it absorbs substances, it sucks them into the inside of the clay particles. Either way, it holds on to the unwanted material until the body removes the clay from the body or the clay is washed off the skin.

Clean bentonite clay boosts immunity. It helps to fight infection. It kills bacteria and viruses.

It seals the leaky gut protecting the gut wall from pesticides, toxins, bacteria, and other chemicals. It helps resolve nausea and vomiting, and it will work as well for constipation as it does for diarrhea. It is also an important tool for chelation of heavy metals and toxin overload.

Bentonite clay helps increase energy and lift brain fog. It helps with headaches, aching joints, and skin problems.

Safety Facts

Pure calcium bentonite clay has a pH of 9.7. When used as a remedy it comes in the form of a very fine and dry powder. It is on the United States Food and Drug Administration's Generally Recognized as Safe (GRAS) list.

Only Use High Quality Bentonite Clay

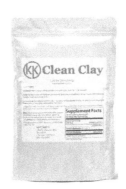

There are many suppliers of bentonite clay. However, many contain lead and other heavy metals – these should be avoided. Also avoid bentonite clay that has been irradiated, washed with alcohol, or otherwise treated.

Kerri recommends using a brand of bentonite clay called Clean Clay™. It has been tested for the presence of heavy metals and toxins. It is truly clean clay.

Methods of Use

Clean Clay can be taken orally or used in a bath.

Instructions for using bentonite clay in a bath are contained in Chapter 6 – in the section, Baths with CD, Salt, or Bentonite Clay.

Mixing Oral Doses of Bentonite Clay

When mixing the bentonite clay in water, do not use a metal object, because metal from the stirrer can be taken up by the clay. It is best to use a glass container with a plastic or wooden spoon to do the mixing.

Does not Remove Minerals or Vitamins

Bentonite clay does not strip minerals or vitamins from the body. Many people believe that when chelators are used, minerals and vitamins are stripped away with the unwanted substances. This is not true.

CHAPTER 4: BLACK SEED OIL

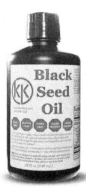

Historical records indicate that black seed oil has been used since ancient times as a natural remedy. It has been said that black seed oil is a cure for everything except death. The oil is made from a specific variety of black cumin seeds that are most often grown in Turkey and India.

Powerful Uses of Black Seed Oil

Black seed oil (BSO) has powerful anti-inflammatory and antioxidant properties. It kills MRSA and the strep that is associated with PANDAS. (PANDAS is Pediatric Autoimmune Neuropsychiatric Disorders Associated with Streptococcal Infections.) PANDAS is one of the conditions common to children on the autism spectrum.

BSO is antifungal, antiparasitic, anticancer, antiasthmatic, and antihistamine. It is great for allergies.

BSO is very important for treating drug resistant pathogens. It is much better than anything else.

It can be used for burns, anti-aging, dandruff, hair growth, etc.

Safety Facts

Black seed oil is a supplement and a food. The USFDA determined that BSO is safe for human consumption. They rated it as GRAS – Generally Recognized as Safe.

Methods of Use

It is very easy to use. You can take it orally as well as using it on every part of your skin. Feel free to apply to the skin as often as needed. It also can be added to an enema or douche. When adding BSO to an enema, you can add an ounce or two to the enema water.

When taken orally, an adult would typically take 1 tablespoon or 15 ml 3 times per day. Children can take half the adult dose. It can be taken with or without food.

Start with a small dose of BSO such as a half teaspoon and increase over time. Some people will work their way up to 2 tablespoons per meal.

I (Kerri) prefer to take BSO with food. I know people who take it without food. You can take it either way.

Provides Omega-3 and Omega-6

A lot of people ask whether they should take omega supplements. We can save money and get better results by taking humic fulvic and black seed oil. Black seed oil provides omega-3 and omega-6 as well as being a killer of pathogens and a healer of all things. It really encourages the body to heal itself, while it is killing parasites and strep. There really is nothing that BSO cannot make better.

CHAPTER 5: WATER PURIFICATION

Public water supplies are not clean. They contain toxic chemicals, pharmaceutical drug residues, heavy metals, and possibly living organisms that escape the disinfection process. For this reason, portable water filtration is extremely important to support long term health.

Impractical Water Filter Options

There are hundreds of water filtering systems on the market today. Some boil water and condense the steam. These distillation units require electricity and are therefore not usable outside the home or during times of electrical interruption.

Two other types of water filters depend on a pressurized water supply from household plumbing to make the process work. Such filters are either reverse osmosis or multi-stage filters. During times when water pressure is low or totally interrupted, these kinds of filters are useless.

Use Anywhere Anytime Water Filters

The most useful and most effective filters are gravity fed systems that allow water to slowly seep through various filtering media to remove heavy metals, pesticides, harmful chemicals and living organisms.

Gravity water filter systems can easily be moved from place to place as needed. They are also less expensive than systems that require electricity and/or pressurized plumbing.

Choosing a Gravity Fed Water Filter

Not all gravity fed water filters are created equal. Mike Adams, the Health Ranger, tested the effectiveness of 12 brands of gravity fed water filters on their ability to remove glyphosate. You can use the link shown below to visit the webpage where he describes the results produced in his laboratory.

Independent laboratory testing results of popular gravity water filters

http://www.waterfilterlabs.com/

Emergency Disinfection of Water

Of course, if all you want to do is disinfect water then you can use 1 drop of CD per liter or quart of water. This will not remove heavy metals, pharmaceutical drugs or other toxins. However, it will kill pathogens and reduce glyphosate levels – two important capacities.

CHAPTER 6: USING CD

Over the years, Kerri has answered tens of thousands of emails about how to use chlorine dioxide (CD). This chapter is intended to provide the information that is most commonly requested by people who are beginning to use CD. This is the information that Kerri would like you to know when you use CD.

People of All Ages Can Use CD

We can all benefit from using CD. It can be used from birth until the end of life.

The correct dose of CD is made by diluting drops of CD in water. It is common to see dosing instructions such as – mix 3 drops of CD in 8 ounces of water and take one ounce of the mixture every hour.

When it is taken orally, it is common to take doses throughout the day. This is because CD is used up by the body in a short period of time.

Kerri reported: During one of my trips to Venezuela, I learned of a 2-month old baby who began suffering from constipation after being vaccinated.

The parents began treating the baby with CD and water. They combined 1 drop of CD with 8 ounces of water, which was divided into 8 doses. Thus, a single dose consisted of 1/8th of a drop of CD mixed in 30 ml (1 oz) of water. The baby was given this dose 8 times a day. They increased the number of drops mixed in water by 1 drop on the next two days until they were mixing 3 drops of CD into 8 ounces of water.

They continued to give 8 doses per day for a couple of weeks. This treatment fixed the gut issues and the baby's gut function returned to normal in only a couple of weeks.

We are able to use CD throughout our lives for treating chronic illnesses like diabetes and autism, as well as for treating things like the common cold.

To maintain good overall health, you can take a dose of CD a few times each week. You only need to take 3 drops of CD mixed in a glass of water a couple of times a week to keep up your good health.

Does CD have Side Effects?

People have asked me if CD, DMSO and other remedies I recommend have "side effects". To answer this, I need to distinguish between the Herxheimer reaction and side effects.

A side effect is a negative consequence of taking a pharmaceutical drug. These are common to most drugs. Side effects can be the appearance of new and undesirable symptoms. Side effects can lead to serious complications and even death. All you need to do is to listen to a drug ad on TV and notice the fast-talking narrator at the end of the commercial as he lists dozens of possible side effects. The list almost always ends with the words, "can cause death."

The natural remedies being discussed in this book do not have side effects. However, with any treatment modality it is possible to have a Herxheimer reaction. The term "Herx" is commonly used as a kind of shorthand term for referring to a Herxheimer reaction.

People who experience a Herx reaction may feel tired or like they are coming down with the flu.

The Herx reaction indicates that a person's body is not able to keep up with eliminating toxins from the body during a course of treatment. Toxins are released by pathogens as they are killed. Our bodies also accumulate numerous kinds of toxins during our lifetime and these toxins can be mobilized during treatment. Regardless of the source of toxins, the body uses its normal mechanisms for removing them.

Responding to a Herxheimer Reaction

When a Herx reaction is experienced, the solution is extremely simple. You can either reduce the treatment dose or increase consumption of water to help the body remove the toxins. The Herx reaction does not last long and is easily corrected by these methods.

The experience of a Herx reaction is an important indicator that the treatment is accomplishing its goals. So, it is actually a positive indicator, though it might cause discomfort for a time.

CD and other Remedies do not cause Harm

Even after many decades of use – the truth is – CD has never harmed anyone regardless of what mainstream media reports have said.

DMSO, another remedy discussed in this book, has been extensively studied by Dr Stanley Jacob since the early 1960s. There has never been anything detrimental observed, though Herx reactions are possible. See the section on DMSO in Chapter 2 for additional information.

Similarly, black seed oil and bentonite clay have been used for thousands of years without negative effects on the body.

Instructions for making CD

Chlorine dioxide is made by mixing two components – sodium chlorite and an acidic activator. People use various activators depending on their personal preferences.

You can use whatever activator you have on hand. I prefer to mix 4% hydrochloric acid (HCl) with a 22.4% sodium chlorite solution when making CD.

You also can use lemon or lime juice to activate the sodium chlorite. Some people believe that the juice should be from fresh lemons or limes.

Citric acid can also be used as the activator. You can use either a 10% or 50% dilution of citric acid.

Mixing the Ingredients

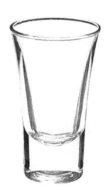

Use a dry shot glass, which is used for drinking alcohol. The shot glass needs to have a rounded (concave) shape bottom inside the glass to force the drops of sodium chlorite and the acid activator to mix together.

Begin by dispensing the desired number of drops of sodium chlorite into the shot glass. For each drop of CD in your desired dose, you use one drop of sodium chlorite plus the required amount of activator to produce one drop of CD.

If you are using 4% HCl as your activator, then add one drop of HCl for each drop of sodium chlorite to make one drop of CD. The activation time is 1 minute. The mixture will turn brown.

If you are using lemon or lime juice, or 10% citric acid as your activator, then add five drops of any one of these acids to each one drop of the sodium chlorite and let activate in the shot glass for 3 minutes. Five drops of activator + one drop of sodium chlorite = one drop of CD.

If you are using 50% citric acid for activation, use one drop of activator for each one drop of sodium chlorite to make one drop of CD. Then let the mixture set for 30-45 seconds.

Best Water to Mix with CD

CD is usually mixed with water before being used, though sometimes it can be taken in capsules. (See below for information about capsules.)

I like to use water that is fluoride free and chlorine free.

It is good to use water that is between 6.8 and 7.1 pH for mixing with CD.

Some people have used bottled waters from Evian or Fiji, which might be good water, yet they are too alkaline for making CD. Alkaline water will decrease the potency of the CD drops when they are added to the water.

Many people only have access to municipal water supplies, which in addition to containing fluoride and chlorine, usually have glyphosate and numerous other chemicals and even trace amounts of pharmaceutical drugs. For this reason, it is very important to filter out these impurities.

There are many types of water filters on the market. I like the gravity fed, ceramic filters that purify the water 99.9% from pretty much everything. See the section on water filters in Chapter 5 for additional information. You also may wish to email me for my recommendation.

You can add CD to drinking water to kill pathogens and to reduce glyphosate levels, but CD does not remove harmful chemicals or pharmaceutical drugs from water. For that level of purification, you will need a good quality gravity fed water filter.

Drinking CD in Water

It is common for people to wonder how much CD they could take during a day. There is no exact answer, but there are guidelines that can help you determine what feels right for you.

I have seen some people comfortably tolerate 13 drops of CD taken in small doses over the day. Other people tolerate 120 drops taken in small hourly doses over a period of 16 hours. The important concept here is the word "tolerate."

To tolerate a dose means you feel good without a detox/Herxheimer reaction. A Herx reaction is nothing more than the detoxification protocol going faster than the body is able to remove the toxins.

If there is a Herx reaction, then you just have to slow down the treatment.

Avoiding a Herx Reaction

I have found that a good method to avoid a Herx reaction is to increase the daily dose in very small increments. If you increase your daily consumption of CD by 1 drop a day and divide that total number of drops into 8 or 16 equal doses, you will almost always avoid a Herx reaction. Just mix the CD with 8 oz or 16 oz of water and take 1 oz 8 or 16 times a day to avoid Herxheimer issues. (See the earlier section in this chapter for additional information about Herxheimer reactions.)

Dosing Patterns

Typically, we take CD hourly throughout the day every day when we have a chronic illness like autism, ADD, ADHD, Lyme, cancer, MS, MRSA, fibromyalgia, Crohn's, high blood pressure, or diabetes.

However, we can also use the hourly dosing for acute situations and discontinue its use after health has been restored.

I always start with 1 drop of CD reduced into 8 or 16 oz of water. I recommend taking 1 oz 8 or 16 times a day depending on the size of the bottle. I would increase daily by 1 drop or as tolerated.

Storage of CD and Water

CD is a gas that mixes easily with water. However, since it is a gas, it will eventually separate from the water and mix with the air.

For best results, consume the CD and water mixture within 72 hours after it has been made. Always keep the mixture in a tightly sealed glass container.

Dosing Patterns with Autism

Recently we have found that people with autism have a faster rate of healing and recovery when they take 22 to 24 doses a day on a 45-minute time schedule – 1 dose every 45 minutes.

This shorter period time between doses is proving to be more successful, I suspect, because it does not give pathogens a chance to multiply.

Weight / Dose Guidelines

Most people are able to tolerate a dose of CD based on their weight.

25-pound child	–	1 drop per hour
50-pound child	–	2 drops per hour
100-pound person	–	3 drops per hour
125-pound person	–	4 drops per hour
150-pound person	–	5 drops per hour
175-pound person	–	6 drops per hour
200-pound person–		7 drops per hour

Bottles for Drinking CD

People use a variety of bottles and jars for drinking CD and water. Recycled glass bottles and glass canning jars are popular. The goal is to find a glass container with a plastic lid that seals tightly and does not leak water or CD.

If you live in a country where glass bottles of VOSS water are sold, then these bottles can be reused as drinking bottles for your daily dose of CD and water – they don't leak. Plastic water bottles are not recommended and bottles with metal lids are not recommended.

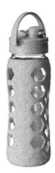

Some people like to use silicon covered water bottles such as those made by LifeFactory (pictured at right).

Quart size canning jars can be used if you do not use the metal lids, but instead buy some plastic replacement lids.

Your choice of bottles should also be geared toward your lifestyle. You want to have a bottle that is easy to use and easy to carry with you when you are on the move. The goal is not so much to find the perfect water bottle as it is to make sure you actually drink your daily dose. When you buy bottles containing food and beverages, you will likely find various options for glass containers with plastic lids that will meet your needs.

Using CD in a Spray Bottle

I, Kerri, make up a spray bottle of CD and water for most everything.

I mix 20 drops of CD for 1 ounce or 30 ml of filtered water.

I spray my fruits and vegetables with CD to disinfect them.

I use CD spray for cleaning my skin, eyes, ears, and mouth.

I spray my toothbrush as well as spraying my gums and teeth. Then, I brush everything in my mouth.

Choosing a Spray Bottle

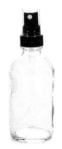

You can use glass or plastic spray bottles for CD and water. They come in a variety of sizes ranging from a few ounces to a quart.

Smaller bottles holding 4 to 8 ounces of liquid are nice because they are easy to transport in a purse or bag. The smaller bottles usually have a non-adjustable mister type spray. You simply push down on the spray head and a very fine mist will be produced.

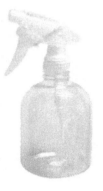

Larger bottles have a trigger type spray head that you pull to release a spray. The spray nozzle can be turned to adjust the fineness of the spray.

Spray bottles can be purchased in clear glass or plastic. There is no advantage for using a blue or amber spray bottle for protecting CD. An advantage for using clear spray bottles is that you can visually monitor the strength of the CD mixture. Over time, the CD will dissipate into the air. As it evaporates, the color will fade – so, you can tell if it has gotten weak. Generally, CD in a spray bottle will be good for use for 7 to 10 days after being made.

Taking CD in Capsules

If you do not like the taste of CD and you are at your full oral dose for CD, then you can put it in capsules to avoid the taste.

New users of CD should not start taking CD in capsules. Doses will need to be broken down into fractional parts of drops in the beginning. For example, you cannot divide a drop into four portions and add a fourth of a drop to a capsule. Drops need to be divided by mixing them into 8 oz, 16 oz, or 24 oz of water to obtain equal dosing.

I do not recommend the use of capsules for most people. However, for adults with autoimmune issues who might be using the CD protocol for Lyme or Multiple Sclerosis over 2 to 4 years, then capsules may make the treatment more tolerable.

Capsules should never be given to non-verbal children on the autism spectrum, because they cannot communicate if a capsule was to get stuck in their throat. It is best to stay with CD in water.

Method for Filling and Taking Capsules

If you are taking 24 drops of CD per day divided into 8 doses, then this means you are taking 3 drops per hour. As an alternative to drinking CD in water every hour, you could take a capsule containing 3 drops of CD every hour.

You can buy empty gelatin capsules at most health food stores or online.

To take CD in a capsule, open an empty gelatin capsule and add 3 drops of sodium chlorite and 3 drops of 4% HCl or an appropriate amount of another activator of your choice. Instructions for using other activators were presented earlier in this chapter.

Assemble the two halves of the capsule immediately after adding the drops. Swallow it with a large glass of water. Do not wait for activation to be complete before swallowing the capsule. Activation will finish while the capsule is in the stomach.

Repeat this process once every hour for 8 hours to take your full daily dose. You will need to assemble a new capsule each hour and not try to make a set of capsules in advance – the capsules will degrade quickly after filling.

Be sure to Drink Water with Capsules

Drinking water is important when taking CD capsules. The minimum amount of water that you want to drink with a capsule containing 3 drops of CD is 3 oz.

Drinking a large glass of water (8 ounces) with each capsule is a better option. If you don't like to drink water, then 3 oz is the minimum.

Nebulizing and Inhaling CD

Place 1 to 3 drops of CD in a large bowl of hot water. Place a large towel over your head and shoulders being sure the towel also covers the bowl. Sit and inhale the steam/CD vapors for 10 minutes. The towel will help contain the steam, which will provide greater opportunity to inhale the CD.

This is actually a very small dose of CD, but it is still helpful. It will help with lung cancer, bronchitis, pneumonia, and head colds.

CD Enemas

One of the reasons that I (Kerri) have been under attack for years is that I recommend enemas. I have been under attack from the outside as well as by people who use CD. Sadly, most people alive today never learned about the benefits of the enema – as a result they fight against this extremely important therapy.

Many alternative healthcare practitioners, however, do understand the long-known truth that health begins in the colon and they do not object to enemas.

Many people who were born after the 1960s and 1970s are not familiar with health and healing treatments like enemas and purges. These were common in the countryside among the wise people who learned from their ancestors.

Enemas have been around for at least 4,000 years. In Egypt there are ancient records of enemas being used. Even the Mayans used the enema. Archeological findings show that the Mayans created clay figures showing the position that a person takes when doing an enema. The clay figure had a happy face.

If you or anyone in your family is not in perfect health, then using enemas may be what is needed to turn the corner of an illness. If the person has any issues or just wants to keep fit, then doing regular enemas will benefit their health.

Frequency for Doing Enemas

You can do enemas daily. Some people do one to four enemas per day. The Gerson cancer program uses five coffee enemas per day to eliminate toxins and to control pain.

Doing an Enema is not Difficult

To take an enema, a person lies down on his side or back, or kneels down with his elbows on the floor. Enema equipment allows warm water with CD to flow into the bowel. The CD kills pathogens such as unhealthy bacteria and parasites. The person then sits on the toilet and releases the water, fecal matter, and parasites.

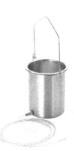

Enema equipment consists of a silicone bag or a small glass or stainless steel bucket that can hold 2 or 3 quarts of liquid. A small flexible silicone hose is connected to the enema bag or bucket, with a silicone tip to insert.

The hose carries the warm water and CD to the anus of the person. A small nozzle or tube at the end of the hose is inserted a couple inches into the anus. Be sure to lubricate the tip with olive or coconut oil. When the clamp on the hose is released, then the water and CD mixture flows into the bowel.

The amount of liquid used in an enema ranges from 1 liter to 5 liters or more. It is best to use filtered water. See the discussion of water filters in Chapter 5 and the information presented earlier in this chapter for additional information about water.

CD/Water Ratio for an Enema

When doing a CD enema, the CD is added to warm water (body temperature) at a rate of 1 drop of CD per 100 ml of water. If we use 1 liter of water, then we add 10 drops of CD. For 2 liters use 20 drops of CD. For 3 liters of water use 30 drops of CD.

Retaining the Enema

When doing a CD enema, it is not necessary to hold the enema in the bowel for a long period of time as is done with coffee enemas. Even after a short time in the colon, the CD kills pathogens and removes biofilm from the bowel.

Constipation and Diarrhea

If constipation is an issue, then I would be doing more than one enema a day. Constipation is a huge issue with cancer and other autoimmune disorders. Even if someone with an autoimmune disorder has diarrhea, CD enemas are still useful.

Constipation and diarrhea are two sides of the same coin. They both indicate gut dysbiosis. If you do not have time to do enemas daily, then do them as often as needed.

Introductory Video on Doing an Enema

There is a great YouTube video by Markus Rothkraz titled "How to do an enema". We like it. We don't like the red rubber bag that he uses, because rubber leaches chemicals into the water. However, his 7-minute explanation on how and why to do enemas is great.

How and Why to do an ENEMA

by Markus Rothkraz

https://www.youtube.com/watch?v=UZEqQlOYXSo
The video is easy to find by using a search engine to look for, "How and Why to do an ENEMA" by Markus Rothkraz."

Some people with MS or cancer do better with colema boards from www.colema.com or www.implantorama.com. This equipment enables a person to repeatedly push much more water into the colon than an enema bag or bucket allows.

Baths with CD, Salt, or Bentonite Clay

These three types of baths serve different purposes.

CD Baths

CD baths are good for a wide variety of ailments. They are useful for shingles, skin rashes, and moles.

CD baths can provide a gentle introduction to the use of CD for people who are highly sensitive to treatments whether natural, alternative, or conventional. These are people who have a hard time starting with oral doses of CD even at the level of 1/16th of a drop per dose.

CD baths can be done daily. They can last as long as a person wants to stay in the tub. You can get the water in your hair, eyes, and ears. Little kids love the baths and can stay in for hours. Kids will swim around in the tub, drink the water, and open their eyes under the water. This is no problem. It is actually better than just sitting and soaking.

You can add 20 to 500 drops of CD into the bath water. A CD bath can be taken as often as desired. ENJOY!

Salt Baths

A salt bath creates an osmotic effect, which draws toxins out of the body. It has the same effect as bathing in the Dead Sea, where people go to bathe for detoxification, rejuvenation, and healing.

We use plain pure salt for the salt bath – not sea salt, Himalayan salt, or Epsom salt – just plain cheap salt. You do not want to use salt that contains anti-caking chemicals. Many types of table salt have these anti-caking agents to prevent it from sticking together in humid weather – avoid these. A good choice is canning salt, which is nothing but salt, NaCl. Be sure to read the ingredient list on the label. It should not list anything other than salt.

Pure salt is inexpensive. If you pay more than $1 (US) per pound or one euro per half kilo, then you are paying too much.

It is suggested to add 9 pounds or 4 kilos of salt to a bathtub of water. The amount of salt is the same for adults and children.

You can soak in the salt bath for as long as you wish – there is no time limit.

A salt bath can be taken daily or as often as you desire.

Bentonite Clay Baths

These are great for heavy metal detoxification.

Add between ¼ of a cup and 1 cup of bentonite clay to the bath water.

Bentonite clay baths can be done daily. You should only spend 10 to 15 minutes in this type of bath.

If you experience hyperactivity or feel unwell during or after a bentonite clay bath, then I would limit the baths to twice a week such as Monday and Friday.

You need to get out of the bentonite clay bath immediately after soaking for 10 to 15 minutes and drain the tub. The heavy metals that were extracted from your body are now in the bath water and it needs to be discarded. Getting out of the tub on time will prevent the metals from being reabsorbed into your body.

For additional information, see the section on bentonite clay in Chapter 3.

Reusing Bath Water

Some people have limited availability of water or it is very expensive. If that is the case for you, and you want to do more than one type of bath on the same day, then follow this bathing sequence.

Do the CD bath first. Then you could add the bentonite clay or the salt to the same water and keep on soaking.

However, do not reverse this order. The CD should not be added afterwards to a salt or bentonite clay bath. This will cause the CD to be neutralized by the salt or clay, and you will not get the benefits of the CD.

CHAPTER 7: SPECIFIC TREATMENTS

Most of the sections in this chapter describe common situations that could happen in our lives at some point. Many conditions could be treated by the conventional medical system. However, historically these conditions were successfully treated at home by friends and family – long before the modern medical care system and Big Pharma existed.

Many of these treatments outperform pharmaceutical drugs. They offer lifesaving alternatives and do so for only pennies.

As mentioned at the beginning of this book, this book does not contain any medical advice. It simply reports the results that people have experienced by using a group of remedies. Kerri is simply describing the use of techniques that will help you on your journey toward better health.

The information presented in this book is not intended or implied to be a substitute for professional medical advice, diagnosis or treatment. All content, including text, graphics, images and information contained in this book is for general information purposes only. Kerri Rivera and John Thomas make no representation and assume no responsibility, legal or otherwise, for the accuracy of information contained in this book. Books are a snapshot in time, and the information this book contains is subject to change as new research becomes available. You are encouraged to confirm any information obtained from or through this book with other sources. Please review all information regarding any medical condition or treatment with your physician. You are ultimately responsible for your own choices surrounding your health and the health of your children.

Bruises and Blood Clots

DMSO is a powerful tool for breaking up blood clots under the skin and inside the body.

Blood Clots under the Skin

A bruise is blood that has clotted under the skin in a localized area.

If you want to promote the healing of common bruising on the skin from life's lumps and bumps or bruising on the face after plastic surgery, then you can simply apply DMSO onto the area. Use it 1 or 2 times per day.

It is extremely important that the skin is clean before applying DMSO. This point cannot be stressed too much. Anything that is on the skin when DMSO is applied will be carried into the body by the DMSO. You don't want to have the DMSO carrying unintentional or toxic substances into the body.

Internal Blood Clots

We also can develop blood clots inside the body. Taking DMSO in oral doses helps with those kinds of clots as well. For example, clots can develop in the lungs.

You can take 8 ml of DMSO mixed in water 3 times a day for internal blood clots. See the section on Strokes in this chapter for additional information about treating blood clots in the body.

My Notes:

Burns

Black seed oil and sodium chlorite are both highly effective treatments for burns.

Sodium chlorite

This is the same sodium chlorite that is used for making chlorine dioxide. In this case the liquid sodium chlorite is used straight from the bottle without mixing with an activator.

You can put the sodium chlorite directly on the burn and wait 2 to 5 minutes before rinsing with cool, clean water. Usually only one or two applications of the sodium chlorite are needed to stop the burning pain. The redness will still fade slowly as the burn heals.

Black Seed Oil

For burns apply black seed oil and keep the skin covered till the burn heals.

My Notes:

Cancer

Cancer can successfully be treated with the CD protocol. Since this book is basically a first aid reference, it does not contain the full protocol. However, there is an important part of the protocol you can use to begin addressing cancer without using the entire protocol.

See the section on Parasites in this chapter for information about parasites and cancer.

Also see the section in this chapter on Chronic Illness and Weakness.

Finally, it is important to understand that CD, DMSO, Black seed oil, and bentonite clay each have properties that can support the overcoming of cancer. See chapters 1 through 4 for information about these remedies.

My Notes:

Chronic Illness and Weakness

If you are very sick with one of the chronic illnesses that are so common today, then you will probably need to use the entire CD protocol to address your situation.

However, as a beginning point, you can start gently by using CD baths and CD oral rinses.

To do an oral rinse with CD, mix 10 drops of CD in 4 to 6 oz of water. Put as much of the mixture in your mouth as you can comfortably hold and keep it in your mouth for 2 to 5 minutes. Repeat this process every hour.

For additional information about using a mouth rinse and mouth care, see the section, Mouth and Throat, in this chapter.

For information about baths, see the section, Baths with CD, Salt, or Bentonite Clay, in Chapter 6: Using CD.

You also might wish to read the section on parasites presented later in this chapter.

My Notes:

Colds

See the section on the Nose, later in this chapter for treatment suggestions.

Constipation and Diarrhea

Please see the section on CD enemas in Chapter 6: Using CD, for information on this topic.

Ears

This treatment works for either acute or chronic ear infections.

Mix 1 drop of CD into 1 oz or 30 ml of filtered water. Use an eye dropper to flood the ear canal with the CD mixture every 15 minutes till the infection is gone. Do not put the eye dropper inside the ear canal – just release the drops so they fall into the ear canal. (See the next section "Eyes" for a picture of an eye dropper.)

You may wish to add a drop of DMSO to the CD and water mixture to help the CD reach the affected area more thoroughly. You can repeat this process as often as you wish.

My Notes:

Eyes

This treatment works great for any eye infection such as acute conjunctivitis (pink eye).

Mix 1 drop of CD in 1 oz or 30 ml of water. Use an eye dropper to put one drop of the mixture in the affected eye every 15 minutes. Do this until the infection is gone.

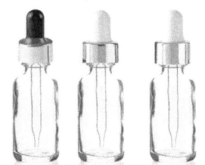

It usually takes 3 to 6 hours to get rid of pink eye. If it is still present after that time, then just keep going.

A pink eye infection can be passed from person to person. So, be sure to wash hands after treating someone. The infected person should use a personal towel in the bathroom until the infection has passed.

My Notes:

Food Poisoning

Food poisoning occurs when we eat food that has an overgrowth of bacteria. This usually happens with food that is left out at room temperature too long. It can also happen from eating raw vegetables that have been watered with unsanitary water or handled by infected people.

If the availability of refrigeration is lost because of electrical service interruptions, then we will all need to eat food shortly after it has been prepared to avoid the possibility of food poisoning.

In many parts of the world, refrigeration is not used, and people develop techniques for keeping food safe. Therefore, it is possible to live without refrigeration.

Sometimes food poisoning happens in restaurants without safe food handling procedures. This may happen with seafood or meat that is not kept cool.

How does it start?

Food poisoning can start with an upset stomach shortly after eating and can progress to vomiting as the body tries to expel the bad food.

How to Respond

If you suspect food poisoning, then mix 3 drops of CD with water and drink that dose every 15 minutes until you feel better.

It is normal for someone experiencing food poisoning to vomit before they take the first dose of CD. If vomiting begins, then still go ahead and take the

CD. The CD will help reduce the nausea. The nausea usually goes away after a few doses of CD.

You might have to do 1 to 3 hours of dosing to resolve the situation. Be sure to drink additional water during this time to avoid dehydration.

My Notes:

Foot Fungus

One of the most difficult and chronic problems facing many people is that of foot fungus. For most of us, our feet spend much of their time in shoes and socks where the feet may stay damp all day long. Fungus thrives in this dark and damp environment.

Ideally, the feet should breathe and be open to the air. Since this is not possible for most of us then we need to resort to a foot fungus protocol to help the feet overcome fungal infections.

Mix coconut, olive or black seed oil and bentonite clay together to make a paste.

Slather the mixture on the feet and toes, and cover with socks. Do this every day before bedtime. Repeat this daily until the foot fungus is gone.

It is important to treat both feet even if the fungus is only observed on one foot. Fungus can spread from the infected foot when it comes into contact with the non-infected foot.

It can be helpful to be sure your shoes have a chance to dry out overnight. If this doesn't happen, then you might want to have more than one pair of shoes and wear them on alternating days to provide for drying time.

My Notes:

Glyphosate Removal from the Body

Even if we eat organic food, we are still being exposed to glyphosate in our food, water, and air.

The Organic Standards from the US Department of Agriculture permit small levels of glyphosate to be present in organic food. This is permitted, because so much of this chemical is being used on farms around the world it can't be controlled. It spreads through the air and through the water. It is in animal feed. It gets into almost every kind of food. It is in most municipal water supplies, and even gets on homegrown vegetables.

Despite the advertising claims that glyphosate (Roundup) is safe, it has been shown in the US courts that it is a carcinogen. It is a very dangerous agricultural chemical. It also interferes with healthy digestion and numerous processes at the cellular level.

Since many of us live in areas where we can't avoid glyphosate exposure, we need to take steps to protect ourselves from being damaged by this chemical.

CD Destroys Glyphosate

Since it is nearly impossible to prevent glyphosate exposure, then it is wise to take steps to destroy the glyphosate that gets into our bodies.

CD should be part of every family's daily water consumption. Stop drinking water taken directly from the kitchen water faucet. Instead set aside water for drinking that has been treated with CD.

Add 1 drop of CD to every liter (or quart) of water that will be consumed by the family. Plan to drink this water every day – not just once in a while, but for every day for the rest of your life.

The CD will remove glyphosate from the body and it will help breakdown the glyphosate that might be in your water.

There are also some gravity fed water filters that remove glyphosate. However, the use of these filters cannot remove the existing burden of glyphosate from the body. See the discussion of water filters in Chapter 5 for additional information.

My Notes:

Hemorrhoids

About half of all people will experience enlarged hemorrhoids at some point in their life. Enlarged hemorrhoids may be accompanied by symptoms in the area of the anus, which include itching, mucus discharge, or pain and bleeding when having a bowel movement with dry hard stool. Many times, people with chronic constipation develop hemorrhoids as a result of prolonged straining when sitting on the toilet.

CD offers relief to people who suffer with hemorrhoids. The beauty of CD is that you cannot do harm – only heal.

CD Enemas

CD enemas are great for helping to shrink and heal hemorrhoids.

You can do an enema with 2 liters (or quarts) of warm water and 20 drops of CD. Do this enema daily. See the section in Chapter 6 on CD enemas for additional information.

CD Irrigation Syringe

If you don't have the time to do an enema or doing an enema is inconvenient, then you can irrigate the inflamed hemorrhoids with a syringe filled with CD and water. To be clear, this is not a hypodermic syringe with a needle. The syringe that is used for this purpose is designed for irrigation. It is large and has a plastic tip that can be inserted in the anus.

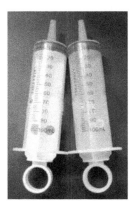

To use this method, mix 2 or 3 drops of CD in 100 ml of water and draw the mixture up into a 100 ml irrigation syringe.

Use the CD filled syringe to irrigate the hemorrhoids when sitting on the toilet. You can do this daily or whenever you experience discomfort. It is important to get the CD water mixture in contact with the affected area.

You can disinfect the tip of the syringe after each use with scalding hot water.

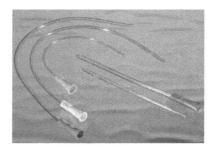

Alternatively, you could connect a catheter (flexible tube) to the end of the syringe and use it to treat the hemorrhoids.

CD Sitz Bath

Another option is to do a CD sitz bath. You can use 20 to 100 drops in the sitz bath. However, few of us have time for much more than the syringe method for hemorrhoid treatment. If water is scarce then the syringe method is best.

My Notes:

Insect Stings and Bug Bites

Treating insect stings involves taking an oral dose of CD and applying CD directly to the skin where you were stung or bit.

Oral Dose of CD

Start by taking an oral dose of CD and water. Mix 6 drops of CD in at least 6 oz of water. Repeat this dose one hour later.

Topical CD

Put 1 drop of CD directly on the sting/bite site, and let it sit for 2 to 5 minutes. Rinse the location with clean, cool water then apply another drop of CD. Repeat this process every 5 to 10 minutes until you experience relief.

Topical Bentonite Clay

If you have some bentonite clay, then take a tablespoon of the clay and add a little water – just enough to create a paste. Apply the paste to the sting/bite site. This will help to pull the toxins out from the skin.

My Notes:

Malaria/Dengue

CD is a fast and simple solution to a serious life-threatening problem plaguing our world. The use of CD could make deaths from malaria and dengue a thing of the past.

Adult Dose: Mix 6 drops of CD in 6 oz (180 ml) of water. Take in the morning. Repeat the same dose the next morning.

Child Dose: Mix 3 drops of CD in 3 oz (90 ml) of water. Give the dose in the morning. Repeat the same dose on the next morning.

That's all there is to the successful treatment of these illnesses!

My Notes:

Mold Exposure

Mold is a big issue for many people today. Oral doses of bentonite clay can be a very helpful treatment.

Adult Dose – Mix bentonite Clay in water and drink the mixture. You can use up to 1 tablespoon of bentonite clay per dose. Take 6 to 10 doses staggered throughout the day. If you plan to take 6 doses, then take a dose every 2 to 3 hours.

If you are already taking oral doses of CD, then you should not take the CD at the same time as the clay. The CD should always be taken 20 to 30 minutes before you take a dose of bentonite clay. This will give the CD time to work in the body before the clay is taken.

Child Dose – Give ¼ to 1 full teaspoon of bentonite clay to the child in water 6 to 10 times a day on the same schedule that is used for an adult.

When mixing the bentonite clay in water, do not use a metal object, because metal from the stirrer can be taken up by the clay. It is best to use a glass container with a plastic or wooden spoon to do the mixing.

My Notes:

Moles

CD and bentonite clay can be used for treating moles.

See the section in Chapter 6 – Baths with CD, Salt, or Bentonite Clay for information about using a bentonite clay bath for moles.

Also see – Skin Tag, Moles, Precancer on Skin, in this chapter for using CD on individual moles.

My Notes:

Mouth and Throat

Oral health is directly connected to our overall physical health and wellbeing.

General Oral Care

Small spray bottles are ideal for using CD in the mouth. Mix 20 drops of CD per every 1 oz (30 ml) of water that you put in a spray bottle.

Spray the CD on your toothbrush as well as spraying it into your throat and on your gums. There is no limit to the amount of CD you can spray. You can swallow the CD after spraying.

You can do this treatment daily as prevention or use it when there is an acute or chronic situation.

Toothache and Gum Abscess

When there is a toothache or gum abscess, you can apply a dab of 99.99% DMSO right on the infected area immediately after brushing. You can reapply the DMSO 4 to 8 times over the course of the day. It is fine to ingest the DMSO.

DMSO is very healthy for us. DMSO is great for so many things, especially in the mouth. It heals the infection as well as reducing the pain and inflammation. You cannot put too much, only too little. So be generous with it.

Sore Throat

For sore throats, coughs, thrush and candida you can use the CD mouth spray and CD mouth gargle.

To use a spray, mix 20 drops of CD in 1 oz of water and add to your spray bottle. Spray in the throat and mouth.

You can also use CD for a mouth rinse and gargle it. Mix 10 drops of CD in a glass of water for this treatment. Put as much of the mixture in your mouth as you can hold. Swish it around in your mouth and/or gargle. You also can just hold the CD in your mouth. The CD will treat the surface area in addition to being absorbed right into your lymphatic system, which will also benefit your overall health.

Use the oral rinse and gargle once or twice a day as part of your routine for brushing your teeth.

My Notes:

Nose

We often feel the first sign of a cold or respiratory problem in the nose. So, it makes sense to treat the nose as soon as nasal stuffiness or irritation is observed.

The nose is treated with an atomizer containing CD and water. A nasal atomizer is a small spray bottle with a tip that is designed for insertion in the nose.

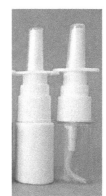

When you squeeze the bottle, a very fine mist of liquid is sprayed up into the nasal passage. To help the spray reach further into the nasal passage, gently inhale through the nose at the same time you squeeze the bottle. There are also atomizers that have a pump mechanism. Either style will work.

To make the nose spray for the atomizer, mix 1 drop of CD with 1 oz (30 ml) of filtered water. Most nasal atomizer bottles are small and may only hold one ounce.

In case of acute infection, you can spray the CD into both sides of the nose every 15 minutes.

The atomizer CD spray bottle can be used for as long as 10 days. Make a new one after that point, if it is still needed. Some people find that it is not necessary to make a second bottle since they feel better after using the CD nasal spray for just one to three days.

You can use the CD nose spray along with oral doses of CD, baths, or enemas to mount an even stronger defense against a cold.

I (Kerri) keep a CD nasal spray bottle on my desk. I use it hourly when I feel the first sign of a winter cold coming on.

The spray is especially useful before airline flights or afterward. It seems that the airlines are recycling more than just air. I usually feel a little tinge of a cold coming on after long flights. So, I make up a CD spray and use it hourly in that situation.

When I feel a cold coming on, I also do an oral rinse with CD as well. It all depends how I feel when the situation is just starting. Anything acute can be nipped in the bud with oral doses of CD, nasal spray, mouth spray, and mouth rinse. See the section Mouth and Throat, in this chapter for additional information.

My Notes:

Pain

DMSO is the best solution for pain, whether acute or chronic. DMSO is curative in nature. It goes far beyond alleviating pain and works to heal source of the pain.

See the overview of DMSO in Chapter 2 for additional information about DMSO and its uses for pain.

My Notes:

Parasites

When a CD enema is used, it is possible to see dead parasites in the enema water when it is released in the toilet. However, a CD enema does not go high enough into the colon to get to all the parasites that might be present. For this reason, other interventions are needed to eliminate parasites from the digestive system.

Parasites release toxic substances into the body and consume nutrients from the food we eat. They steal our vitality and can harm our ability to think. They can even give us cravings to eat food that the parasites want, even when we know those foods are unhealthy for us.

Mebendazole, Albendazole, and Fenbendazole are pharmaceutical drugs that have been developed for treating parasites in animals. However, they are equally effective in humans.

Reports now show that Mebendazole and Fenbendazole also have a powerful benefit that goes far beyond killing parasites. These medications also have the ability to eliminate cancer cells from the human body. They destroy tumors at the stem cell level while being basically harmless to human health.

All three of these medications are available online without a prescription. Do not be put off by the fact that you will find them listed online at pet pharmacies. Humans can and do consume these kinds of drugs.

These three drugs are not to be taken at the same time – use them separately as indicated. You may wish to consult with Kerri to obtain additional information about using these treatments as part of a more extensive protocol.

Mebendazole

Parasite Treatment – people weighing over 100 lbs (45 kg) should take 200 mg of Mebendazole twice a day with meals.

Cancer treatment – people can take 400 mg of Mebendazole twice a day until the cancer is gone.

Fenbendazole

For cancer treatment – take 1 gram of Fenbendazole per day for 3 consecutive days. Then take 4 days off. It can be taken with or without food at any time of the day. Follow this weekly pattern for up to 14 weeks or until the cancer is in remission.

Albendazole

For systemic parasites – adults should take 400 mg of Albendazole twice a day with meals. It can be taken for short period of a few days or for a week or more. Children should take half the adult dose.

The recommended protocol is to take Albendazole for 6 weeks at the dose mentioned above, then take 2 weeks off. Follow this with 6 more weeks of Albendazole at 1 mg per pound of body weight. Take this dose twice a day at mealtime.

There is synergy in using Albendazole with CD. Together, they do a better job of eradicating parasites.

My Notes:

Pets

We give CD to pets primarily based on their weight.

For general health and protection of our pets we can add 1 to 6 drops of CD to the pet's water bowl each day.

If the pet gets sick, then we can give 1 to 5 drops of CD as an oral dose every hour or so. It all depends on weight. You can err on the side of caution of you are unsure.

Pretty much any pet between 20 to 100 lbs (10 to 45 kilos) can be given 1 drop of CD mixed in water every hour with a large plastic syringe designed for irrigating or feeding.

It is very important to accompany the drops of CD with the appropriate amount of water. Every drop of CD must be mixed in 1 oz (30 ml) of water. If you have a large dog, around 100 pounds, then give the dog 3 drops of CD mixed with 3 oz of water in the syringe.

Be sure to make clean water available to pets so they can drink as much as they wish for flushing their body of toxins.

You can add 1 to 5 drops of DMSO to the CD/water mixture in the syringe.

You can also give DMSO to a pet without the CD. You would still use a syringe and water. Depending on the weight of the animal you can give 1 ml to 8 ml of DMSO at various times of the day.

DMSO works against pathogens as well as cancer. It is great for driving CD or anything else deep into the body of a pet.

DMSO also can be used topically to clean skin or fur. Topical and oral doses of DMSO are great for pets that suffer from arthritis. DMSO is very inexpensive as well as very effective. It's good for the whole family.

My Notes:

Rashes

See the section in Chapter 6 – Baths with CD, Salt, or Bentonite Clay for using a bentonite clay bath for rashes.

Shingles

See the section in Chapter 6 – Baths with CD, Salt, or Bentinite Clay for using a bentonite clay bath for shingles.

Sores on Skin that don't Heal

You can apply black seed oil to sores that don't heal. It is a great aid to healing.

My Notes:

Skin Tags, Moles, Precancerous Growths

I (Kerri) had a weird "freckle" over my eyebrow. It was a light color and then became darker with time. Finally, it became much darker and started to look like it had dry skin on it.

I went to the dermatologist and he told me it was precancerous and to put some cream on it. The cream was a chemotherapy type product, and I wanted no part of it.

So, I went home and activated 2 drops of CD in a shot glass and dipped the tip of a cotton swab in the pure undiluted CD. I put the CD right on the freckle and held it there for a couple of minutes. I immediately repeated the treatment a second time. On the next day, I repeated the treatment a third time.

By day 3 the spot hurt like a burn. It turned red and after a few days turned into a scab. Shortly after that the scab fell off.

The skin underneath the scab was new and pink. After a couple of months, the area looked just like the rest of the skin on my face. Mission accomplished. I would do this for any weird skin thing.

I also put black seed oil on the burn at bedtime. It helped to heal the burn faster, and is good for any burn, intentional or not.

I could have added 1 or 2 drops of DMSO to the 2 drops of pure CD to drive the CD into the skin more deeply. I did not do that in this case.

I do enjoy spraying a mixture of CD, DMSO, and water on my skin to enhance the effects of the CD to obtain its added benefits.

My Notes:

Spiders – Poisonous Bites

If you are somewhere where there is no emergency help for a poisonous spider bite, then you should not panic – you have an intervention in your pharmacy of the future first aid kit.

Start by taking oral doses of CD every hour. Each hourly dose should contain 1 to 3 drops of CD mixed in 1 to 3 oz of water. Do this every hour all day long.

You can also make a paste from activated charcoal, bentonite clay, and a small amount of water. Apply the paste to the affected area.

The paste will draw out the toxins from the skin. If you have CD spray, then spray it on the affected area when it becomes dry.

My Notes:

Stroke

DMSO is a powerful treatment for dissolving blood clots such as those that cause a stroke. A stroke is characterized by a weakened ability to move parts of the body. It could be the partial impairment of certain muscles of the face or the loss of the ability to move an arm or leg.

The first signs of a stroke could be the drooping of one side of the face or an eye, slurred or incoherent speech, arm or leg weakness, or the inability to lift the arms over the head. It can be seen in an inability to stick out the tongue and move it from one side of the mouth to the other.

Treatment should start immediately at the first appearance of symptoms. Treatment can also be undertaken by people who had a stroke several weeks or months ago. There is no detrimental effect from treating an old stroke. However, the sooner you start taking DMSO after a stroke the better chance you will have for a full recovery.

DMSO Dosing for a new Stroke

During the first hour – Mix 2 tablespoons (30 ml) of DMSO in 4 oz (120 ml) of water. Drink this dose every 15 minutes for the first hour.

For the rest of the day – mix 1 Tablespoon (15 ml) of DMSO in 2 oz (60 ml) of water. Drink this dose every 15 minutes for the rest of the day.

DMSO Dosing for an Old Stroke

If you had a stroke in the past then it is a good idea to take 1 Tablespoon (15 ml) of DMSO mixed in 2 oz (15 ml) of water twice a day indefinitely.

Technique for Mixing DMSO in Water

Never measure DMSO in a plastic spoon or mix DMSO with water in a plastic cup, because it can leach toxic chemicals from the plastic. Always use a glass container.

My Notes:

Teeth and Gums

See the section, Mouth and Throat, in this chapter for information on this topic.

Vaginal Care and Yeast

CD douches are the best treatment for vaginal care. They can be used to help women "freshen up," and to respond to the presence of a chronic illness such as a tumor, cyst, or a nagging yeast infection.

In order to kill pathogens in the vagina, it is necessary to get the CD mixture in contact with as much tissue area as possible and to maintain the contact for up to 2 minutes. CD kills pathogens immediately on contact, yet, sometimes it can take up to 2 minutes for that contact to be completely achieved.

To prepare the CD douche, mix 1 drop of CD for every 10 ml of water that will be used for the douche.

You can use an irrigation syringe to place the CD into the vagina. Fill a 60 ml or 100 ml syringe with the CD and water mixture. Use 6 drops of CD in a 60 ml syringe and 10 drops of CD in a 100 ml syringe.

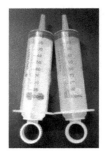

For best results, hold the douche for 2 minutes. Of course, you can do longer or shorter if you wish.

For the water to stay in the vagina, you need to lie down and elevate your hips above your shoulders. The ideal position is to lie on the bathroom floor with the shoulders on the floor. Place the heels of your feet on the top edge of the tub so that you can easily lift and hold your hips in the air while you are holding the douche.

The CD douche should not be done during the week of menstruation.

People with breast cancer will benefit from using the CD douche.

The CD douche can be used daily until the problem you are treating is gone. There is no limit to the frequency of use. The only detail is that you should use 1 drop of CD per 10 ml water.

Some women like to do CD douches as a part of their routine healthcare. They do these douches periodically even when they are not having a specific health concern.

My Notes:

CHAPTER 8: AVOIDING POISONS

If there is a major breakdown in social infrastructure and an economic collapse, then we will all face many new challenges for keeping ourselves healthy. For example, ensuring that we have clean drinking water, nontoxic food, and simple remedies for treating our health needs will be essential for long-term survival.

There will also be a hidden poison that we would do well to avoid during difficult times. Unfortunately, this poison is already with us today, and it is already weakening us and making us more vulnerable to modern illnesses. When the collapse comes, it will raise our stress levels even higher in ways we can't totally predict.

The stressor I (John) am about to discuss is produced by wireless technology. This energetic poison is a burden that surrounds us, penetrating our DNA, and suppressing our vitality.

The electronic devices that we use and the supporting systems that enable them to function are a major long-term health risk. I don't expect wireless technology to fail during times of collapse, because these systems are part of a social control system and propaganda mill that will be needed to control us when things get difficult.

I have been researching the risks associated with devices such as smartphones, Wi-Fi, and smart meters during the past five years or so, and will summarize some of the steps you can take to reduce the stress on your body today and in the future.

High stress is a burden that helps illness progress within us. Reducing the stress that technology places on our body and mind will help us build up vitality and avoid illness. This is important at any time in our lives, but when the great crash comes, it will give us the ability to cope with great hardship.

We will have greater mental and physical strength and will be better able to focus our efforts on what is truly important.

5G Warning

Background

Telecom companies are quickly installing a new generation of cellular service called 5G. This will be the fifth generation of wireless phone service. It will use much shorter wave lengths than have been used in the past. This non-ionizing radiation in the millimeter frequency band will put much more stress on all forms of life especially human life.

There will be 5G small cell towers located throughout all urban areas. The towers will be placed on top of utility poles and all manner of public infrastructure such as bus shelters, schools, and other public buildings. The towers will be located 500 feet to 1,000 feet apart on every city street in cities – small and large – throughout the world.

In addition, several companies have already begun to deploy satellites that will beam a similar 5G type service over every square foot of the Earth.

This new 5G technology has not been studied for safety. Concerned scientists have warned the World Health Organization that research shows that we should have serious concern about exposure to 5G radiation and increased cancer risk, cellular stress, increase in free radicals, genetic damage, changes in the reproductive system, learning and memory deficits, and neurological disorders. [1] As I see it, 5G will cause an intensification of chronic illnesses of all kinds.

Directed Energy Beam Technology

There are two large differences between 5G and earlier generations of wireless communication. The first was already mentioned – the use of much shorter millimeter frequency waves. The second is that the new technology will use directed energy beam technology, which is also called beam steering technology.

These new 5G small cell towers and the new 5G smartphones will use phased array antennas to send and receive information by means of energy beams. You can think of these beams of energy as being similar to invisible laser beams. They will travel from a 5G cell tower right to your smartphone. Your phone and the tower will send and receive information through this beam of energy. As you move, the beam will follow you and constantly expose you to non-ionizing radiation.

The directed energy beam will pass through objects including your body and head in order to get to your phone. Even if you are not talking or browsing the internet, the 5G beams will be present and stand ready for immediate use. One consequence of this is that your location will always be known by your cellular service provider and anyone with whom they share that information.

Protecting Yourself from 5G Radiation

One of the important steps you can take is to minimize the amount of time that your 5G phone is turned on. I know that for many people this will require a serious change in how they use their phone. Remember that if you keep your phone turned on and carry it on your body, there will be highly charged millimeter energy beams passing through your body all day long. This radiation will be much more intense than previous generations of phones regardless of what telecom companies might tell us.

Second, don't bring the 5G phone (or any other cellphone) into your bedroom at night. When charging it, keep the phone as far away as possible from people and pets.

Finally, don't fall for the advertising hype that insists everyone should and must have a 5G phone. These new phones will use existing 4G networks until the 5G infrastructure is fully implemented. 4G will still be available for a considerable number of years. So, just keep using your 4G phone. If it dies, then just buy the latest generation 4G phone and don't step up to the "newest and greatest" 5G equipment.

Wi-Fi and Other Wireless Devices

Wi-Fi is commonly used to provide wireless connections between computers and the internet. It broadcasts large amounts of microwave radiation throughout most homes and office buildings. It is used in hotels, coffee shops, and anywhere large numbers of people gather with their laptop computers.

If you have a Wi-Fi router in your home, then you will sleep better and be healthier if you turn it off at night.

An even healthier solution is to replace the Wi-Fi unit with a wired router and DSL cables. This will provide maximum protection from the microwave radiation produced by Wi-Fi units.

Similarly, stop using wireless baby monitors and cordless home phones. Replace them with corded options to avoid the constant broadcast of unhealthy frequencies into the environment.

Smart Meters and Smart Appliances

Smart meters are used to transmit wireless data to the electric power company about the electricity you use in your home. In some locations, there are also smart meters that measure water and natural gas use. These devices produce a constant stream of pulsing energy transmissions throughout homes and offices, which suppresses the immune system and even alters heart rhythm.

In addition, new generation appliances such as refrigerators and dishwashers interact with these smart meters and wirelessly report their activities to the smart meter. The result of this is a constant high level of frequency pollution throughout the home and surrounding environment.

In most locations, customers can request to have the smart meters removed and replaced with older style analog meters. You might have to pay a monthly surcharge to protect your family from the frequencies these devices produce, but the health benefits will be worth the cost.

When buying appliances, do extra research to be sure that they are not smart meter compatible. Some appliances may be able to interact with smart meters even if they don't proudly say it in the product advertising.

Minimize the Effects of Non-ionizing Radiation

One of the biggest threats to our health from 5G and even earlier generation cellular services is the burden of heavy metals that we carry around with us in our bodies. Mercury, lead, aluminum, cadmium, barium, and other metals act as microscopic antennas. If we have metals in our bodies, and most of us do, then our bodies will attract non-ionizing radiation from cellular transmissions of all types.

To minimize the damage from these transmissions, we should take steps to expel the heavy metals from our bodies as soon as possible.

There are three approaches that work together to bind and remove the metals from our bodies.

Use EDTA with Selenium and Minerals™

EDTA is a chelator – it removes metals. When taking this formula, begin by taking 2 drops of the solution 3 times a day before meals. Increase the dose over time until a maximum of 20 to 30 drops is taken 3 times a day. It may be added to spring water if extra minerals are desired.

Use Zeolite

The natural mineral Zeolite has been proven to absorb toxins, free radicals, and heavy metals from the body. It also boosts the immune system without side effects. This mineral will balance the body's pH.

Use Clean Bentonite Clay

See the description of bentonite clay in Chapter 3. Also see the section, Baths with CD, Salt, or Bentonite Clay, in Chapter 6.

Reference

[1] "'Flying Blind' with 5G," The Alliance for Natural Health, 1/2/2020. https://anh-usa.org/flying-blind-with-5g/

CHAPTER 9: BE PREPARED

For those of us who contemplate the signs of social and economic decline, we have serious concerns about the stability of the future.

We wonder whether a day will be coming soon when life as we have known it will crumble and we will have to find new ways to take care of ourselves and our families.

Among the many changes we will likely face is the probable loss of the modern medical care system. Our access to it might disappear or the thousands of pharmaceutical drugs that it depends upon may no longer be available.

In response, we will need to have our own personal pharmacy of nontoxic remedies that can be easily stored for a long period of time. This "pharmacy of the future" needs to be easily transported and easily used in primitive living conditions.

Preppers Pharmacy

If the worst-case scenario happens and there is a collapse of society as we know it, then it would be advantageous to have a stock of empty glass bottles, dropper bottles, and spray bottles in order to be able to give people prepared solutions of CD and other remedies.

Cash money may no longer be used, and remedies could be exchanged for food or other things that you and your family may need.

It may be wise to keep a good stock of the sodium chlorite and the activator on hand for long-term future use. It stores well in a cool, dark place for years.

Your Bugout/Camping Bag

Some people prepare for the great collapse by having a bugout bag packed and ready to go for the day when it is necessary to leave their homes and migrate to some other location. Others may not be quite so well prepared, but they do wilderness camping and want to have a proper selection of first aid supplies beyond bandages for cuts and sprains.

Regardless of how you prepare for the future, these are the essential items you would want to have with you.

CD kit

DMSO

Bentonite clay

Black seed oil

Gravity water filter

If you are a prepper, then it would be a good idea to have large quantities of the above items for bartering or helping others. You will need to have large quantities of empty dropper bottles, spray bottles, sealable bottles, and atomizer bottles if possible.

Additionally, to protect yourself from the most extreme effects of 5G technology, it would be useful to have a supply of EDTA and zeolite, which were discussed in Chapter 8: Avoiding Poisons, which can be used along with bentonite clay to detoxify yourself from heavy metals.

Water Disinfection Equipment

If you want to disinfect your drinking water whether or not you are taking CD as a treatment modality for a specific illness, you can add 1 drop of CD to a liter of water. There are approximately 4 liters in a gallon.

Water filters are an essential part of being prepared for a time of great social upheaval. Water filters were discussed in Chapter 5.

Fasting by Necessity or for Health

Many of us have not experienced a shortage of food because of famine or because the grocery stores are out of stock. It is quite possible that future events could leave us without a steady supply of food. Stocking up on nonperishable food is one possible solution to this potential problem, but even then, circumstances might unfold where we are separated from our food supply.

If we are camping or traveling to a safer location, and food becomes unavailable, then it will be useful to know how to fast.

Fasting for Health

Fasting can also be a treatment strategy for many health conditions. It can be especially useful for situations where previous healing strategies don't seem to be working.

It is not unusual to see adults with various illnesses such as MS or Crohn's disease, who have tried a myriad of diets and supplements. Despite the effort and tens of thousands of dollars spent on supplement-based protocols, they remain sick. In these cases, sometimes fasting can be the key to recovering health.

When people begin fasting, they will begin to see a reduction of symptoms. Fasting is effective and free!

I (Kerri) am a huge fan of Cole Robinson, the snake diet founder. His work is very useful for going more deeply into this topic. He has an extensive set of instructional materials on his Facebook groups, YouTube channels, and on Instagram.

This type of fasting is not intermittent fasting where food is eaten every day during a small window of time. The fasting that is being described here involves not eating for 24 to 72 hours to promote healing.

It is important to maintain your mineral levels while fasting. Kerri recommends using humic fulvic solution for supplying minerals while fasting.

Cole Robinson recommends something called snake juice when fasting. To make his snake juice, combine a liter of water with ½ tsp of potassium chlorite (NO SALT brand) and ¼ tsp of Himalayan salt. Optionally, you can add up to 2 tablespoons of apple cider vinegar to the mix. Plain water can be consumed, though he prefers that people just drink his snake juice formula.

What Happens to the Body When Fasting?

This summary was adapted from the work of Cole Robinson.

After 12 hours of fasting, the healing begins. It starts after the last meal has been digested and the digestive system goes to sleep. At this point, the levels of HGH (human growth hormone) begin to increase. Glucagon is released to balance blood sugars.

At 16 hours, the body starts fat burning.

At 18 hours HGH starts to skyrocket.

At 24 hours of fasting, autophagy begins and ketones begin to be released into the bloodstream.

Autophagy is a natural process by which our cells disassemble and remove their dysfunctional components. It can be thought of as taking out the trash. There will be a reduction of inflammation and improved immune system functioning at this point, and the process of aging slows down. Healthy immune system cells will hunt out dead and diseased cells and consume them – cancerous cells are destroyed, and infectious particles and toxins are removed. Fasting does not cause the loss of muscle at this point.

At 36 hours of fasting, the autophagy increases 300%. Ketone levels increase and ketosis can begin. Ketosis is a safe and healthy condition suitable for sustaining life. Ketosis should not be confused with ketoacidosis, which is a life-threatening condition experienced by type 1 diabetics.

At 48 hours of fasting, autophagy increases another 30%. There will be an immune system reset and regeneration, and there will be increased reductions in the inflammatory response.

After 48 to 72 hours of fasting, the glycogen stores will be depleted. The body will use ketones for energy.

24-Hour Fasting and Eating Cycle

If you want to fast for health and you do not have any extra weight to lose, then you can eat one nutrient-dense low carb meal once every 24 hours and still have excellent results.

Nutrition for Optimal Health

The very best way we can be prepared for any eventuality is to be in optimal health. Nutrition is the cornerstone of the foundation for vibrant health. One of the most important keys to restoring health, attaining and maintaining optimal strength is to eat a nutrient dense ketogenic diet made up of whole natural foods. It should have adequate protein (about 20%), the majority of calories from fat (75-80%), and very low or no calories from carbohydrates.

It should include foods from animal sources, including plenty of fats, and low starch vegetables. Fats from fruits such as coconut, palm and olive are permissible. Animal fats are very important because they contain the fat-soluble vitamins A, D3, and K2. These vitamins ensure that minerals are put in our bones and teeth and not in our arteries. They help our immune system deal with infections.

The optimal diet should omit sugars, refined grains and seed oils. These industrial foods deplete the body of vitamins and minerals. They also cause many other disruptions in the normal body metabolism, including obesity and Type 2 diabetes.

People are finding that a ketogenic diet is very satisfying and easy to maintain because it doesn't cause the blood sugar swings and cravings that come from eating carbohydrate foods. Your energy will be stable and available when needed.

CHAPTER 10: FINAL THOUGHTS

It is hoped that the information in this book will be complete enough to help you respond to dozens of health concerns. Of course, there were many topics that we did not include, but we believe that the principles that were described for using CD, DMSO, bentonite clay, black seed oil, and water filtering will enable you to creatively apply solutions to situations we did not discuss.

We hope and pray that God will accompany you on your healing journey and be a comforting and wise presence as you respond to illness and seek improved health. You are not alone in your journey!

Please remember that Kerri Rivera is available to answer questions by email if you need further clarification of the topics presented here, or you just don't know where to begin your journey toward greater health.

Kerri Rivera's Email:

kerri@kerririvera.com